The MIND Diet and Intermittent Fasting

A guide to using intermittent fasting to boost the effectiveness of the MIND Diet.

COPYRIGHT © 2023

All rights reserved.

The information contained in this book is based on the author's research and experience. While the author has made every effort to provide accurate and up-to-date information, errors and omissions may occur. The author and publisher assume no responsibility for any errors or omissions or for any actions taken based on the information contained in this book.

The information contained in this book is provided "as is," without warranty of any kind, express or implied, including but not limited to the warranties of merchantability, fitness for a particular purpose, or non-infringement. In no event shall the author or publisher be liable for any claim, damages, or other liability, whether in an action of contract, tort, or otherwise, arising from, out of, or in connection with the book or the use or other dealings in the book.

TABLE OF CONTENTS

INTRODUCTION

In the ever-evolving landscape of health and nutrition, where trends come and go like fleeting whispers, two dietary strategies have emerged as giants in their respective domains. The MIND diet, renowned for its brain-boosting potential, and intermittent fasting, celebrated for its metabolic and longevity benefits, stand as pillars of wellness in our modern era.

Imagine, for a moment, the fusion of these two nutritional powerhouses — a dynamic synergy where the health of your mind and body converge. It's a concept that goes beyond mere nourishment; it's a paradigm shift in the way we approach our well-being. In this comprehensive guide, we will unveil the extraordinary potential of combining intermittent fasting with the MIND diet to create a harmonious symphony of health, where your cognitive vitality meets the vigor of disciplined fasting.

The MIND diet, short for "Mediterranean-DASH Diet Intervention for Neurodegenerative Delay," was designed with the noble goal of reducing the risk of cognitive decline and Alzheimer's disease. It draws inspiration from the Mediterranean and DASH (Dietary Approaches to Stop

Hypertension) diets, both celebrated for their heart-healthy properties. The MIND diet's unique twist lies in its emphasis on foods proven to support brain health, such as leafy greens, berries, nuts, and whole grains. With a focus on nourishing your gray matter, the MIND diet is a dietary framework that aspires to keep your mental faculties sharp and your cognitive well-being intact.

In the other corner of this nutritional arena stands intermittent fasting (IF), a practice that transcends traditional eating patterns. Instead of dwelling on what you eat, IF is concerned with when you eat. It's a rhythm of feast and fast, a dance of nourishment and restraint that has been practiced by cultures and faiths around the world for centuries. More than just a fad, intermittent fasting has been recognized by the scientific community for its myriad health benefits. It can aid in weight management, improve metabolic health, and even extend lifespan. IF is a potent tool for enhancing physical vitality and resilience.

So, what happens when we marry the mindful principles of the MIND diet with the disciplined cadence of intermittent fasting? The answer is a symphony of well-being—a harmonious balance between physical health and cognitive acuity. In this guide, we will delve deep into the science behind this remarkable fusion, exploring the mechanisms through which intermittent fasting can amplify the effectiveness of the MIND diet.

But our journey does not stop at scientific theory. We are here to equip you with practical knowledge and actionable steps to integrate these dietary strategies into your daily life. Whether you are a newcomer to both the MIND diet and intermittent fasting or a seasoned practitioner of one or the other, this guide has something to offer.

PART ONE

WHAT IS THE MIND DIET?

The MIND diet is a dietary pattern designed to promote brain health and reduce the risk of cognitive decline, particularly Alzheimer's disease. The term "MIND" stands for "Mediterranean-DASH Diet Intervention for Neurodegenerative Delay." It combines elements of two well-known dietary approaches: the Mediterranean diet and the DASH (Dietary Approaches to Stop Hypertension) diet, while also focusing on specific foods and nutrients believed to have a positive impact on brain function.

The MIND diet emphasizes foods that are rich in nutrients thought to support cognitive health and protect against neurodegenerative diseases. These foods include:

• Leafy Greens: Vegetables like spinach, kale, and collard greens are rich in vitamins, minerals, and antioxidants that are beneficial for the brain.

• Berries: Blueberries, strawberries, and other berries are packed with antioxidants, particularly flavonoids, which may help protect brain cells from damage.

• Nuts: Almonds, walnuts, and other nuts are a source of healthy fats, vitamins, and minerals that can support brain health.

• Whole Grains: Foods like whole wheat, oats, and brown rice provide a steady supply of energy to the brain and contain important nutrients like fiber, B vitamins, and antioxidants.

• Fatty Fish: Fish like salmon, mackerel, and sardines are high in omega-3 fatty acids, which are essential for brain function and may reduce the risk of cognitive decline.

• Olive Oil: Olive oil, especially extra-virgin olive oil, is a staple in the Mediterranean diet and is associated with various health benefits, including brain health.

• Poultry: Lean sources of poultry like chicken and turkey are included in moderation.

• Beans and Legumes: Beans, lentils, and other legumes provide fiber, protein, and essential nutrients for brain health.

• Wine (in moderation): Red wine, in moderation, is allowed due to its potential antioxidant properties, though excessive alcohol consumption is discouraged.

• Herbs and Spices: Foods like turmeric and cinnamon, known for their anti-inflammatory properties, are encouraged.

The MIND diet also recommends limiting or avoiding certain foods believed to be less conducive to brain health, including:

• Red Meat: Consumption of red meat is limited on the MIND diet.

• Butter and Margarine: High-fat dairy products and trans fats are discouraged.

• Cheese: High-fat cheese intake is limited.

• Fried and Fast Foods: These are to be consumed sparingly or avoided.

• Pastries and Sweets: Limit sugary snacks and desserts.

• Processed Foods: Highly processed foods with added sugars and unhealthy fats should be minimized.

• Whole Milk: Low-fat or skim milk is recommended over whole milk.

The MIND diet is not only about the specific foods you eat but also the overall dietary pattern. It encourages a balanced and varied diet that includes plenty of fruits and vegetables, whole grains, and healthy fats while limiting processed and unhealthy foods.

Research suggests that following the MIND diet may reduce the risk of Alzheimer's disease and cognitive decline. While it is not a guaranteed prevention or treatment for these conditions, adopting a MIND diet-inspired approach to eating can contribute to better brain health and overall well-being.

WHAT ARE THE FUNDAMENTALS OF THE MIND DIET

The MIND diet (Mediterranean-DASH Diet Intervention for Neurodegenerative Delay) emphasizes specific foods that are associated with brain health and is designed to reduce the risk of cognitive decline and neurodegenerative diseases, such as Alzheimer's disease. The diet combines elements from two well-known dietary patterns: the Mediterranean diet and the DASH (Dietary Approaches to Stop Hypertension) diet. Here are the fundamentals of the MIND diet:

• Leafy Greens: Leafy green vegetables like spinach, kale, and collard greens are rich in nutrients like folate and vitamin K, which have been linked to improved cognitive function. These greens are a staple of the MIND diet and are encouraged to be consumed regularly.

• Berries: Berries, especially blueberries, are known for their high levels of antioxidants, such as flavonoids. These antioxidants can help protect brain cells from oxidative stress and inflammation, potentially reducing the risk of cognitive decline.

• Nuts: Nuts are a source of healthy fats, including omega-3 fatty acids and antioxidants, which can benefit brain health. Almonds, walnuts, and other nuts are included in the MIND diet.

• Whole Grains: Whole grains like brown rice, whole wheat bread, quinoa, and oats provide a steady supply of glucose to the brain, offering sustained energy. They are encouraged as part of the diet.

• Fatty Fish: Fatty fish such as salmon, mackerel, and sardines are rich in omega-3 fatty acids, particularly DHA (docosahexaenoic acid), which is essential for brain function. Consumption of these fish is recommended.

• Olive Oil: Extra virgin olive oil, a key component of the Mediterranean diet, is a source of monounsaturated fats and antioxidants. It has been associated with reduced cognitive decline and is the preferred cooking oil in the MIND diet.

• Poultry: Lean sources of protein, such as chicken and turkey, are allowed in moderation.

• Beans and Legumes: Beans and legumes like lentils, chickpeas, and black beans are rich in fiber, protein, and various nutrients beneficial for overall health, including brain health.

• Wine (in moderation): Moderate consumption of red wine is permitted due to its resveratrol content, which has been linked to certain cognitive benefits. However, it's important to consume alcohol in moderation, as excessive alcohol intake can have detrimental effects on health.

• Limiting Red Meat, Butter, Margarine, Cheese, Pastries, and Sweets: These items are discouraged or should be consumed sparingly, as they have been associated with a higher risk of cognitive decline and various health issues.

The MIND diet also encourages other healthy lifestyle habits, including:

• Regular Exercise: Physical activity is an essential component of overall health and brain function.

• Staying Socially Active: Engaging in social activities and maintaining a strong social network can benefit cognitive health.

• Maintaining a Healthy Body Weight: Obesity is a risk factor for cognitive decline, so maintaining a healthy weight is emphasized.

What makes the MIND diet unique is its specific focus on foods that have been scientifically linked to brain health. While it is not a guarantee against cognitive decline, adopting the MIND diet can be a valuable dietary strategy to support cognitive well-being as we age.

WHAT IS INTERMITTENT FASTING?

Intermittent Fasting (IF) is an eating pattern that alternates between periods of fasting (not eating or consuming very few calories) and periods of eating. Unlike traditional diets that focus on what you eat, intermittent fasting primarily focuses on when you eat. It does not prescribe specific foods but rather provides a structured approach to meal timing.

There are several popular methods of intermittent fasting, each with its own fasting and eating windows. Some of the common IF methods include:

• 16/8 Method: This method involves fasting for 16 hours each day and restricting eating to an 8-hour window. For example, you might eat between 12:00 PM and 8:00 PM and fast from 8:00 PM to 12:00 PM the next day. These fasting days are often referred to as "fasting" days, while the other days are "feasting" days.

• 5:2 Diet: In this approach, you eat normally for five days of the week and restrict your calorie intake to around 500-600 calories on the other two non-consecutive days.

• Eat-Stop-Eat: This method involves fasting for a full 24 hours once or twice a week. For example, you might fast from dinner one day to dinner the next day.

• Alternate-Day Fasting (ADF): With ADF, you alternate between days of regular eating and days of fasting or consuming very few calories.

• The Warrior Diet: In this approach, you fast for most of the day and consume all your calories within a short eating window, typically 4 hours.

• OMAD (One Meal a Day): With OMAD, you eat only one meal per day, typically within a one-hour window, and fast for the remaining 23 hours.

Intermittent fasting has gained popularity in recent years due to its potential health benefits, including:

• Weight Loss: By reducing the time available for eating, IF can create a calorie deficit, leading to weight loss.

• Improved Insulin Sensitivity: Fasting periods can enhance insulin sensitivity and help regulate blood sugar levels.

• Cellular Repair: Fasting triggers autophagy, a cellular process that removes damaged components and supports cellular repair.

• Heart Health: IF can lead to improved cardiovascular health by reducing risk factors like high blood pressure, cholesterol, and triglycerides.

• Longevity: Some animal studies suggest that intermittent fasting may extend lifespan, although more research is needed in humans.

• Brain Health: Fasting may support brain health by promoting the production of brain-derived neurotrophic factor (BDNF), which is associated with cognitive function.

It's important to note that intermittent fasting is not suitable for everyone, and its effectiveness can vary from person to person. Individuals with certain medical conditions, pregnant or breastfeeding women, and those with a history of eating disorders should approach intermittent fasting with caution and consult with a healthcare professional before starting.

Also, it's crucial to focus on the quality of the food consumed during eating periods and ensure that nutrient needs are met to maintain overall health while practicing intermittent fasting.

BENEFITS OF THE MIND DIET

The MIND diet, designed specifically to support brain health and reduce the risk of cognitive decline and neurodegenerative diseases like Alzheimer's, offers several potential benefits:

• Reduced Risk of Cognitive Decline: One of the primary goals of the MIND diet is to reduce the risk of cognitive decline as we age. Numerous studies have shown that adherence to the MIND diet is associated with a lower risk of cognitive impairment and Alzheimer's disease.

• Improved Brain Health: The MIND diet is rich in foods that are scientifically linked to better brain health. Nutrient-dense foods like leafy greens, berries, and fatty fish provide essential vitamins, antioxidants, and omega-3 fatty acids that support cognitive function.

• Heart Health: The MIND diet incorporates many heart-healthy components, such as olive oil, whole grains, and nuts. These foods can help lower the risk of cardiovascular diseases, which in turn can benefit brain health by improving blood flow to the brain.

• Weight Management: The MIND diet encourages the consumption of nutrient-dense, fiber-rich foods, which can help with weight management. Maintaining a healthy weight is associated with a lower risk of cognitive decline.

• Reduced Inflammation: The MIND diet's focus on foods rich in antioxidants and anti-inflammatory properties can help reduce inflammation in the body. Chronic inflammation has been linked to various diseases, including those affecting the brain.

• Stabilized Blood Sugar Levels: Whole grains and foods with a low glycemic index in the MIND diet can help stabilize blood sugar levels. This can reduce the risk of type 2 diabetes, which is associated with an increased risk of cognitive decline.

• Protection Against Oxidative Stress: Berries, nuts, and leafy greens are packed with antioxidants that help protect brain cells from oxidative stress, a process associated with aging and cognitive decline.

• Improved Mood and Mental Well-being: Some components of the MIND diet, such as omega-3 fatty acids from fatty fish, have been linked to improved mood and reduced risk of depression.

• Longevity: While more research is needed, some studies suggest that adherence to the MIND diet may be associated with increased longevity, potentially due to its positive effects on overall health.

• Flexibility and Sustainability: The MIND diet is flexible and can be adapted to various dietary preferences, making it a sustainable long-term dietary approach for many individuals.

It's important to note that while the MIND diet offers many potential benefits for brain health, it is not a guaranteed preventive measure against cognitive decline or neurodegenerative diseases. Genetics, lifestyle factors, and other variables also play significant roles in brain health. Nonetheless, the MIND diet provides a structured and science-backed approach to nourishing the brain and supporting overall well-being.

BENEFITS OF INTERMITTENT FASTING

Intermittent fasting offers a range of potential benefits, supported by scientific research and anecdotal evidence. Here are some of the notable advantages associated with intermittent fasting:

• Weight Management: Intermittent fasting can lead to reduced calorie intake, which often results in weight loss. This is because it helps regulate eating patterns and promotes a calorie deficit, particularly in time-restricted eating methods.

• Improved Metabolic Health: Intermittent fasting has been linked to improved insulin sensitivity, which helps regulate blood sugar levels. It may also lead to better metabolic health, potentially reducing the risk of type 2 diabetes.

• Cellular Repair and Autophagy: Fasting triggers a process called autophagy, in which the body removes damaged cells and regenerates new, healthy ones. This can support cellular repair and may contribute to longevity.

• Heart Health: Some studies suggest that intermittent fasting can lead to improved heart health by reducing blood pressure, cholesterol levels, and inflammation, all of which are risk factors for cardiovascular disease.

• Enhanced Cognitive Function: Intermittent fasting may stimulate the production of brain-derived neurotrophic factor (BDNF), a protein associated with cognitive function, learning, and memory.

• Reduced Inflammation: Intermittent fasting has been shown to reduce markers of inflammation, which are associated with chronic diseases like heart disease, cancer, and neurodegenerative disorders.

• Improved Blood Sugar Control: Intermittent fasting may help stabilize blood sugar levels by enhancing insulin sensitivity and reducing insulin resistance.

• Weight Loss without Muscle Loss: Unlike some diets that may lead to muscle loss along with fat loss, intermittent fasting tends to preserve lean muscle mass while promoting fat loss.

• Longevity and Anti-Aging Effects: Animal studies have suggested that intermittent fasting may extend lifespan and delay the aging process, though more research is needed in humans.

• Better Cellular Health: Intermittent fasting may stimulate autophagy, a process that helps the body remove damaged cells and regenerate new, healthier ones. This supports overall cellular health.

• Potential Cancer Benefits: Some studies in animals and limited human research suggest that intermittent fasting may have potential anti-cancer effects, although more research is needed.

• Simplicity and Convenience: Intermittent fasting is relatively straightforward and doesn't require complicated meal planning or special foods. This can make it a convenient approach to healthy eating.

It's important to note that while intermittent fasting can offer numerous benefits, it may not be suitable for everyone. Individuals with certain medical conditions, pregnant or breastfeeding women, and those with a history of eating disorders should consult with a healthcare provider before starting an intermittent fasting regimen. Additionally, the quality of food consumed during eating periods is crucial. Prioritizing nutrient-dense, balanced meals is essential for overall health and well-being.

SCIENTIFIC BACKGROUND OF THE MIND DIET

The MIND diet is a dietary pattern that has gained attention for its potential to support brain health and reduce the risk of cognitive decline and neurodegenerative diseases, such as Alzheimer's disease. While it draws inspiration from the Mediterranean and DASH (Dietary Approaches to Stop Hypertension) diets, it has its own unique focus on foods that have been scientifically linked to cognitive function. Here is a brief overview of the scientific background of the MIND diet:

1. Dietary Components and Brain Health:

The MIND diet emphasizes specific foods that have shown a positive association with cognitive function and brain health in scientific studies. These include leafy greens, berries, nuts, whole grains, fish, and olive oil.

2. Antioxidants and Anti-Inflammatory Compounds:

Many of the foods recommended in the MIND diet are rich in antioxidants and anti-inflammatory compounds. Antioxidants help protect brain cells from oxidative stress and damage, while reducing inflammation is believed to be beneficial for cognitive function.

3. Omega-3 Fatty Acids:

Fatty fish, such as salmon and mackerel, are staples of the MIND diet due to their high content of omega-3 fatty acids. Omega-3s have been linked to improved brain function and a reduced risk of cognitive decline.

4. Berries and Cognitive Function:

The MIND diet places particular emphasis on berries, especially blueberries, which are known for their high levels of antioxidants, particularly flavonoids. Studies have suggested that regular consumption of berries is associated with better cognitive performance.

5. Leafy Greens and Cognitive Health:

Leafy greens like spinach and kale are rich in nutrients such as folate and vitamin K, which are believed to support cognitive health. Some research has shown that higher intake of leafy greens is associated with a reduced risk of cognitive decline.

6. Nuts and Healthy Fats:

Nuts are included in the MIND diet due to their content of healthy fats, fiber, and various nutrients. Healthy fats, such as those found in nuts and olive oil, are considered beneficial for brain health.

7. Whole Grains and Steady Energy:

Whole grains, another key component of the MIND diet, provide a steady source of energy to the brain. They help regulate blood sugar levels and may reduce the risk of cognitive decline.

8. Limiting Red and Processed Meats:

The MIND diet advises limiting the consumption of red meat and processed meats, which are associated with an increased risk of cognitive decline. It recommends lean sources of protein instead.

9. Wine in Moderation:

The MIND diet allows for moderate consumption of red wine. This is due to the presence of resveratrol, a compound found in wine, which has been linked to certain cognitive benefits. However, excessive alcohol consumption is discouraged.

10. Long-Term Cognitive Health:

The MIND diet is not a quick-fix solution but a long-term approach to promoting cognitive health. It encourages sustained adherence to these dietary principles over time.

While research on the MIND diet is ongoing, several studies have suggested that adherence to this dietary pattern is associated with a reduced risk of cognitive decline and neurodegencrative diseases. However, further research is needed to confirm these findings and better understand the precise mechanisms by which the MIND diet may support brain health.

Intermittent fasting is a dietary pattern that involves alternating periods of eating with periods of fasting. Its scientific background encompasses a range of physiological and cellular responses that can have significant impacts on overall health. Here are some key aspects of the scientific background of intermittent fasting:

1. Insulin Sensitivity and Blood Sugar Regulation:

Intermittent fasting has been shown to improve insulin sensitivity, which is the body's ability to respond effectively to insulin and regulate blood sugar levels. This can help reduce the risk of insulin resistance and type 2 diabetes.

2. Cellular Repair and Autophagy:

Fasting triggers a process called autophagy, in which the body cleans out damaged cells and regenerates new, healthy ones. This process supports cellular repair and may contribute to longevity.

3. Hormone Regulation:

During fasting periods, levels of certain hormones change. For example, levels of norepinephrine (noradrenaline) and human growth hormone increase, which can lead to increased fat burning and improved muscle preservation.

4. Weight Management and Fat Loss:

Intermittent fasting can lead to reduced calorie intake, as it sets specific time windows for eating. This often results in weight loss and reduced body fat percentage, which is beneficial for overall health.

5. Reduced Inflammation:

Some studies have suggested that intermittent fasting may lead to a reduction in inflammatory markers. Chronic inflammation is associated with various chronic diseases, including heart disease and neurodegenerative conditions.

6. Heart Health:

Intermittent fasting may lead to improved heart health by reducing risk factors such as blood pressure, cholesterol levels, and inflammation.

7. Cognitive Function and Neuroprotection:

Fasting may stimulate the production of brain-derived neurotrophic factor (BDNF), a protein associated with cognitive function, learning, and memory. Additionally, intermittent fasting has shown potential in protecting against neurodegenerative diseases.

8. Gene Expression and Longevity:

Some animal studies have suggested that intermittent fasting may lead to changes in gene expression related to longevity and cellular health, potentially extending lifespan.

9. Improved Blood Lipid Profile:

Intermittent fasting may lead to improvements in lipid profiles, including reduced levels of triglycerides and LDL cholesterol.

10. Potential Cancer Benefits:

Some animal studies and limited human research suggest that intermittent fasting may have potential anti-cancer effects, though more research is needed.

11. Autonomic Nervous System Balance:

Intermittent fasting may help balance the autonomic nervous system, which regulates involuntary functions like heart rate, blood pressure, and digestion.

12. Mitochondrial Function:

Fasting may enhance mitochondrial function, which is crucial for cellular energy production and overall metabolic health.

While intermittent fasting can offer numerous benefits, it's important to approach it with caution and consult with a healthcare provider, especially for individuals with certain medical conditions or those taking medications. Additionally, it's crucial to prioritize nutrient-dense, balanced meals during eating periods to support overall health and well-being.

HOW THE MIND DIET AND INTERMITTENT FASTING COMPLEMENT EACH OTHER

The MIND diet and intermittent fasting are two distinct dietary approaches, each with its unique set of benefits. However, when combined strategically, they can complement each other and create a synergy that may be particularly beneficial for brain health. Here's how these two dietary strategies work together to support cognitive well-being:

1. Enhanced Nutrient Intake during Eating Windows:

Intermittent fasting involves specific time periods for eating, which can be used to maximize nutrient intake. When individuals break their fasts during the eating window, they have the opportunity to consume foods rich in brain-boosting nutrients, as emphasized by the MIND diet.

For example, during the eating window, individuals can prioritize leafy greens, berries, nuts, fatty fish, and whole grains — key components of the MIND diet. This ensures that they receive essential vitamins, antioxidants, and omega-3 fatty acids that support cognitive function.

2. Improved Insulin Sensitivity and Blood Sugar Control:

Intermittent fasting has been shown to enhance insulin sensitivity, helping regulate blood sugar levels more effectively. This is particularly relevant to brain health because fluctuations in blood sugar can negatively impact cognitive function.

By stabilizing blood sugar levels through fasting, individuals can complement the MIND diet's emphasis on low-glycemic, nutrient-dense foods that support brain health.

3. Autophagy and Cellular Repair:

Fasting periods in intermittent fasting trigger autophagy—a cellular process that removes damaged cells and promotes cellular repair. This process can complement the MIND diet's focus on protecting brain cells from damage. By engaging in intermittent fasting, individuals may enhance the brain's natural ability to repair and regenerate cells, potentially providing additional neuroprotection.

4. Weight Management and Cognitive Benefits:

Intermittent fasting can aid in weight management, which is crucial for brain health. Excess weight, especially visceral fat, is associated with cognitive decline. By facilitating weight loss and fat reduction, intermittent fasting complements the MIND diet's goals of maintaining a healthy body weight for improved cognitive function.

5. Anti-Inflammatory Effects:

Both the MIND diet and intermittent fasting have shown potential anti-inflammatory effects. Chronic inflammation is linked to cognitive decline and neurodegenerative diseases. The combination of these two dietary strategies may provide a more comprehensive approach to reducing inflammation and supporting brain health.

6. Cognitive Clarity and Mental Acuity:

Intermittent fasting has been associated with enhanced mental clarity and focus during fasting periods. This heightened cognitive state can be leveraged for tasks requiring concentration and creativity. Aligning fasting windows with cognitive tasks or work periods can maximize productivity and align with the MIND diet's goals of improving cognitive function.

7. Neuroprotection:

The combination of intermittent fasting and the MIND diet can act as a powerful shield against neurodegenerative diseases. It fortifies the brain against oxidative stress, inflammation, and cellular damage. The synergistic effect of these dietary strategies may provide robust neuroprotection, reducing the risk of cognitive decline.

In summary, intermittent fasting and the MIND diet can complement each other to create a holistic approach to brain health. While intermittent fasting regulates eating patterns, stabilizes blood sugar, and promotes cellular repair, the MIND diet provides a foundation of brain-boosting nutrients. Together, they can enhance cognitive function, reduce the risk of neurodegenerative diseases, and support overall well-being. However, it's essential to consult with a healthcare provider or nutritionist before embarking on a combined dietary approach, especially if you have underlying health conditions or specific dietary needs.

BENEFITS OF COMBINING INTERMITTENT FASTING WITH THE MIND DIET

Combining intermittent fasting with the MIND diet can create a powerful synergy that enhances brain health and overall well-being. Here are the benefits of integrating these two dietary approaches:

1. Enhanced Cognitive Function:

Intermittent Fasting: Fasting triggers the production of brain-derived neurotrophic factor (BDNF), a protein associated with improved cognitive function, learning, and memory.

MIND Diet: The MIND diet emphasizes foods rich in antioxidants, omega-3 fatty acids, and other nutrients known to support cognitive function.

2. Reduced Risk of Cognitive Decline:

MIND Diet: The MIND diet is specifically designed to reduce the risk of cognitive decline and neurodegenerative diseases like Alzheimer's.

Intermittent Fasting: Fasting periods promote autophagy, a process that helps remove damaged brain cells, potentially reducing the risk of neurodegenerative diseases.

3. Improved Insulin Sensitivity and Blood Sugar Control:

Intermittent Fasting: Intermittent fasting improves insulin sensitivity and helps regulate blood sugar levels, reducing the risk of insulin resistance and type 2 diabetes.

MIND Diet: The MIND diet emphasizes whole grains, fruits, and vegetables with a low glycemic index, which further supports stable blood sugar levels.

4. Weight Management and Metabolic Health:

MIND Diet: The MIND diet promotes weight management through the consumption of nutrient-dense, low-calorie foods.

Intermittent Fasting: Intermittent fasting encourages the use of stored fat for energy, leading to improved metabolic health and reduced risk factors for cognitive decline.

5. Antioxidant and Anti-Inflammatory Effects:

MIND Diet: The MIND diet's emphasis on fruits, vegetables, and berries provides a rich source of antioxidants that protect brain cells from oxidative stress and inflammation.

Intermittent Fasting: Fasting reduces inflammation and oxidative stress, contributing to a healthier brain environment.

6. Neuroprotection and Cellular Repair:

MIND Diet: Specific components in the MIND diet, such as omega-3 fatty acids, folate, and antioxidants, offer neuroprotective benefits.

Intermittent Fasting: Fasting triggers autophagy, a process that helps remove damaged cells and regenerate new, healthy ones, which supports overall cellular health, including brain cells.

7. Simplicity and Sustainability:

MIND Diet: The MIND diet is a practical, balanced, and sustainable dietary pattern that can be followed long-term.

Intermittent Fasting: Intermittent fasting is a straightforward and accessible approach to eating that does not require complex meal planning.

8. Longevity and Anti-Aging Effects:

Intermittent Fasting: Some studies suggest that intermittent fasting may extend lifespan and delay the aging process, potentially due to its effects on cellular repair and metabolic health.

By integrating intermittent fasting with the MIND diet, individuals can tap into the combined benefits of both approaches, creating a holistic and powerful strategy for promoting brain health, reducing the risk of cognitive decline, and supporting overall well-being. However, it's important to consult with a healthcare provider before making significant changes to your diet or fasting regimen, especially if you have underlying health conditions.

POTENTIAL RISK OR CHALLENGES OF COMBINING INTERMITTENT FASTING WITH THE MIND DIET

Combining intermittent fasting with the MIND diet can offer numerous benefits, but it may also present some potential risks and challenges, depending on individual circumstances and how these dietary approaches are implemented. Here are some considerations:

1. Nutrient Deficiency:

Challenge: Combining two dietary approaches may inadvertently lead to nutrient deficiencies if not carefully planned. Extended fasting periods, especially when combined with restrictive diets like the MIND diet, may limit nutrient intake.

Solution: Ensure that you are getting a wide variety of nutrient-dense foods during your eating windows. Pay particular attention to essential nutrients like vitamins, minerals, and protein. Consider consulting with a registered dietitian for personalized guidance.

2. Hunger and Discomfort:

Challenge: Fasting periods can be challenging, especially if you are not used to extended periods without food. You may experience hunger, irritability, and discomfort.

Solution: Start with shorter fasting windows and gradually extend them to allow your body to adapt. Stay hydrated, and consider incorporating small, balanced snacks during fasting periods if necessary.

3. Blood Sugar Fluctuations:

Risk: Combining intermittent fasting with the MIND diet may lead to blood sugar fluctuations, particularly if fasting periods are extended. This can be problematic for individuals with diabetes or those prone to hypoglycemia (low blood sugar).

Solution: If you have diabetes or blood sugar issues, consult with a healthcare provider or registered dietitian before implementing intermittent fasting. They can help you develop a safe and effective plan that meets your specific needs.

4. Medication Interaction:

Risk: Some medications, such as those for diabetes or blood pressure, may need to be adjusted when following an intermittent fasting regimen. Combining fasting with the MIND diet can affect how medications work.

Solution: Consult with your healthcare provider before making any changes to your medication regimen. They can provide guidance on how to adapt your medication schedule to accommodate fasting.

5. Eating Disorders and Psychological Impact:

Risk: Intermittent fasting may trigger or exacerbate eating disorders or unhealthy relationships with food in some individuals. Combining it with dietary restrictions from the MIND diet may increase the risk.

Solution: Individuals with a history of eating disorders or those who are susceptible to them should approach intermittent fasting cautiously or avoid it altogether. Seek guidance from a mental health professional or registered dietitian if needed.

6. Social and Lifestyle Challenges:

Challenge: Fasting schedules can sometimes conflict with social or work-related obligations, making it difficult to maintain a consistent routine.

Solution: Plan your fasting and eating windows around your lifestyle as much as possible. Communicate with family, friends, and coworkers about your dietary choices to help create a supportive environment.

7. Lack of Long-Term Research:

Challenge: While there is growing evidence supporting the individual benefits of intermittent fasting and the MIND diet, there is limited long-term research on the safety and effectiveness of combining these two approaches.

Solution: Be cautious and monitor your health closely. If you experience any adverse effects, consider adjusting your approach or seeking professional guidance.

It's crucial to remember that not everyone will experience the same outcomes when combining intermittent fasting with the MIND diet. What works well for one person may not work as effectively for another. Individual factors, including age, health status, and lifestyle, should be taken into account when considering these dietary approaches. Consulting with a healthcare provider or registered dietitian before making significant dietary changes is advisable, especially if you have underlying health conditions or concerns. They can help you create a safe and personalized plan that aligns with your health goals.

FOODS TO EAT WHEN COMBINING INTERMITTENT FASTING WITH THE MIND DIET

When combining intermittent fasting with the MIND diet, it's important to focus on nutrient-dense foods that support brain health and provide sustained energy throughout the fasting period. Here are some recommended foods to include in your eating window:

• Leafy Greens: Spinach, kale, collard greens, and Swiss chard are rich in antioxidants, vitamins, and minerals that support brain health.

• Berries: Blueberries, strawberries, and raspberries are high in antioxidants, particularly flavonoids, which are beneficial for cognitive function.

• Fatty Fish: Salmon, mackerel, sardines, and trout are rich sources of omega-3 fatty acids, which have been linked to improved brain health and cognitive function.

• Nuts and Seeds: Almonds, walnuts, chia seeds, and flaxseeds provide healthy fats, fiber, and a range of nutrients beneficial for brain function.

• Whole Grains: Brown rice, quinoa, whole wheat bread, and oatmeal offer complex carbohydrates, providing sustained energy and essential nutrients for brain health.

• Lean Poultry: Chicken and turkey are good sources of lean protein, which is essential for overall health, including brain function.

• Legumes and Beans: Lentils, chickpeas, black beans, and kidney beans are rich in protein, fiber, and various nutrients that support cognitive function.

• Olive Oil: Extra virgin olive oil is a source of monounsaturated fats and antioxidants, which are beneficial for brain health.

• Avocado: Avocado is a nutrient-dense fruit that provides healthy fats, fiber, and various vitamins and minerals beneficial for cognitive function.

• Colorful Vegetables: Bell peppers, carrots, tomatoes, and other colorful vegetables are rich in antioxidants and provide a range of nutrients that support brain health.

• Eggs: Eggs are a good source of protein, as well as nutrients like choline, which is important for brain health.

• Herbs and Spices: Herbs like rosemary, turmeric, and cinnamon have been associated with cognitive benefits and can be used to add flavor and nutrients to meals.

• Low-Fat Dairy or Dairy Alternatives: Yogurt, milk, and cheese (in moderation) provide calcium, protein, and other essential nutrients for brain health.

• Lean Red Meat (in moderation): Lean cuts of red meat like lean beef or lamb provide essential nutrients like iron and vitamin B12, which support overall health.

• Water and Herbal Teas: Staying well-hydrated is important for overall health, including brain function. Water and herbal teas can help keep you hydrated.

Remember to focus on whole, minimally processed foods and aim for a balanced intake of macronutrients (carbohydrates, proteins, and fats) to support overall health. Additionally, consult with a healthcare provider or registered dietitian to ensure that your dietary choices align with your individual health goals and needs.

When combining intermittent fasting with the MIND diet, it's important to avoid or limit foods that may have a negative impact on brain health and overall well-being. Here are foods to avoid or limit:

• Sugary and Processed Foods: Avoid sugary snacks, candies, soda, and processed foods high in added sugars. Excessive sugar intake is associated with cognitive decline.

• Trans Fats: Limit or avoid foods containing trans fats, such as partially hydrogenated oils and many fried and baked goods. Trans fats are linked to inflammation and cognitive impairment.

• Red and Processed Meats: Reduce the consumption of red meat, especially processed meats like bacon, sausages, and hot dogs. High red meat intake has been associated with cognitive decline.

• High-Sodium Foods: Limit foods that are high in sodium, such as processed meats, canned soups, and fast food.

Excessive salt intake can lead to high blood pressure, which is detrimental to brain health.

• Fast Food and Fried Foods: Minimize fast food and fried foods, which are typically high in unhealthy fats, sodium, and calories that can negatively impact cognitive function.

• Highly Processed Snacks: Avoid highly processed snack foods like potato chips, crackers, and packaged cookies, which often contain unhealthy fats and additives.

• Artificial Sweeteners: Limit the use of artificial sweeteners like aspartame and sucralose, as their long-term effects on brain health are still being studied.

• Alcohol in Excess: While moderate alcohol consumption, especially red wine, is allowed on the MIND diet, excessive alcohol intake can have detrimental effects on brain health and should be limited.

• Butter and Margarine: Minimize the use of butter and margarine, which are high in saturated and trans fats. Choose healthier cooking oils like olive oil instead.

• Excessive Caffeine: Limit excessive caffeine consumption, as it can lead to sleep disturbances and negatively impact cognitive function if consumed in large amounts.

• Processed Cheese and Full-Fat Dairy (in excess): While some dairy is allowed on the MIND diet, high consumption of full-fat dairy products and processed cheeses may not be ideal for brain health due to their saturated fat content.

• Highly Refined Grains: Avoid highly refined grains like white bread, white rice, and sugary cereals. Opt for whole grains, which provide more nutrients and sustained energy.

• Excessive Calorie Consumption: Avoid overeating during eating windows. Even healthy foods can be detrimental if consumed in excessive amounts, leading to weight gain and potential cognitive impairment.

It's essential to maintain a balanced and mindful approach to eating during both fasting and eating windows. Prioritize whole, nutrient-dense foods that align with the principles of the MIND diet to support brain health and overall well-being. Additionally, staying well-hydrated with water and herbal teas can help you maintain cognitive function and energy levels during fasting periods.

A STEP-BY-STEP GUIDANCE ON HOW TO IMPLEMENT INTERMITTENT FASTING WITHIN THE FRAMEWORK OF THE MIND DIET

Implementing intermittent fasting within the framework of the MIND diet can be a beneficial approach for brain health and overall well-being. Here's a step-by-step guide on how to do it:

Step 1: Understand the MIND Diet Principles

Familiarize yourself with the principles of the MIND diet, which emphasizes brain-boosting foods such as leafy greens, berries, nuts, whole grains, and fatty fish, while limiting processed and sugary foods.

Step 2: Consult with a Healthcare Provider

Before starting any fasting regimen, consult with a healthcare provider or registered dietitian, especially if you have underlying health conditions or take medications. They can provide personalized guidance and ensure that intermittent fasting is safe for you.

Step 3: Choose an Intermittent Fasting Method

Select an intermittent fasting method that aligns with your lifestyle and preferences. Common methods include the 16/8 method (16 hours fasting, 8 hours eating), 5:2 diet (eating normally for five days, fasting or consuming very few calories for two non-consecutive days), or the Eat-Stop-Eat method (fasting for a full 24 hours once or twice a week).

Step 4: Establish Your Eating Window

Determine your eating window, which is the period during which you'll consume all your calories. Ensure that this eating window aligns with the principles of the MIND diet and includes brain-boosting foods.

Step 5: Plan Balanced Meals

During your eating window, plan well-balanced meals that incorporate MIND diet principles. Include foods like:

• Leafy greens (spinach, kale, collard greens)

• Berries (blueberries, strawberries)

- Nuts (almonds, walnuts)

- Fatty fish (salmon, mackerel)

- Whole grains (brown rice, quinoa)

- Lean poultry (chicken, turkey)

- Beans and legumes (lentils, chickpeas)

- Olive oil (use as a primary cooking oil)

Limit or avoid foods that are not MIND-diet-friendly, such as processed meats, sugary snacks, and high-sodium foods.

Step 6: Stay Hydrated

Drink plenty of water during fasting periods to stay hydrated. Herbal teas or black coffee (without added sugar or cream) are often acceptable during fasting hours.

Step 7: Monitor Your Eating Habits

Pay attention to portion sizes and mindful eating practices during your eating window to prevent overeating. Focus on nutrient-dense, whole foods.

Step 8: Track Your Progress

Keep a journal to monitor your progress, including how you feel, your energy levels, and any changes in weight or cognitive function. This can help you assess the effectiveness of the combined approach.

Step 9: Adapt and Modify

Be flexible and open to adjustments. If you find that a particular fasting schedule or meal plan isn't working for you, consider modifying it to better fit your needs and lifestyle.

Step 10: Prioritize Nutrient Density

Ensure that you prioritize nutrient-dense foods that support brain health within your eating window. The MIND diet's emphasis on antioxidants, omega-3 fatty acids, and other nutrients remains crucial.

Step 11: Maintain Social Engagement

While fasting, continue to engage socially and adapt your fasting schedule to accommodate social events when necessary.

Schedule regular check-ins with your healthcare provider or registered dietitian to assess your progress, address any concerns, and make adjustments as needed.

Remember that the combined approach of intermittent fasting and the MIND diet is a long-term strategy for brain health and overall well-being. It's important to prioritize safety, sustainability, and personalization in your journey to optimize cognitive health through these dietary practices.

MEAL TIMING

Meal timing is a critical aspect of intermittent fasting (IF) and can vary depending on the specific IF method you choose. The timing of your meals and fasting periods will dictate when you eat and when you abstain from food. Here's a breakdown of meal timing for some common intermittent fasting methods:

1. 16/8 Method (Time-Restricted Eating):

Fasting Period: Typically, this method involves fasting for 16 hours each day, including the overnight fast while you sleep.

Eating Window: The eating window is 8 hours long. For example, you might eat from 12:00 PM to 8:00 PM or 10:00 AM to 6:00 PM.

Meals: During the eating window, you can have 2-3 meals and possibly a snack or two, depending on your preferences.

2. 5:2 Diet:

Fasting Days: On fasting days, you restrict calorie intake to around 500-600 calories, typically consumed in two small meals or snacks.

Regular Days: On regular days, you can eat normally without calorie restrictions.

3. Eat-Stop-Eat:

Fasting Period: With this method, you fast for a full 24 hours once or twice a week.

Meals: On fasting days, you do not eat any solid food. You may consume non-caloric beverages like water, herbal tea, or black coffee (without added sugar or cream).

4. Alternate-Day Fasting (ADF):

Fasting Days: On fasting days, you consume very few calories or none at all.

Eating Days: On eating days, you can eat normally, with no calorie restrictions.

5. Warrior Diet:

Fasting Period: This method involves fasting during the day and consuming one large meal in the evening.

Fasting Phase: You fast for 20 hours.

Eating Window: The eating window is 4 hours, typically in the evening.

Meal: During the eating window, you have one large meal.

6. Spontaneous Meal Skipping:

This is a less structured form of IF where you skip meals whenever you feel like it. Some people might skip breakfast or lunch on occasion.

When planning your meal timing for intermittent fasting:

• Stay hydrated during fasting periods with water, herbal tea, or black coffee (without added sugar or cream).

• Focus on nutrient-dense, balanced meals during your eating windows to meet your nutritional needs.

• Listen to your body's hunger and fullness cues, and adjust your eating and fasting windows if needed to ensure the approach is sustainable and comfortable for you.

It's important to choose an intermittent fasting method and meal timing schedule that align with your lifestyle, preferences, and health goals. Consulting with a healthcare provider or registered dietitian can provide personalized guidance to ensure your chosen approach is safe and effective for you.

PORTION CONTROL

Portion control is important when practicing intermittent fasting (IF) to ensure that you make the most of your eating windows while still managing your calorie intake effectively. Here are some tips for portion control during intermittent fasting:

• Use Smaller Plates and Bowls: Eating from smaller dishes can create the illusion of a larger portion, helping you feel more satisfied with less food.

• Measure Your Food: Use measuring cups, a kitchen scale, or your hand (e.g., a palm-sized portion of protein) to gauge portion sizes accurately.

• Prioritize Protein: Include lean sources of protein in your meals. Protein helps you feel full and satisfied, making it easier to control portion sizes.

• Fill Half Your Plate with Vegetables: Vegetables are low in calories and high in fiber, providing bulk to your meals without adding excessive calories.

• Mindful Eating: Pay attention to portion sizes and practice mindful eating during your eating windows to prevent overeating. Focus on nutrient-dense, whole foods to maximize the benefits of your meals.

• Plan Balanced Meals: Aim for balanced meals that include a variety of food groups. A typical plate might consist of half vegetables, a quarter protein, and a quarter whole grains or starchy vegetables.

• Avoid Distractions: Eating while distracted, such as watching TV or working at your desk, can lead to overeating. Focus on your meal and savor the experience.

• Pre-Portion Snacks: If you have snacks during your eating window, pre-portion them into small containers or bags to prevent mindless snacking.

• Stay Hydrated: Drink water before and during your meals. Sometimes, thirst can be mistaken for hunger.

• Listen to Your Body: Pay attention to your body's hunger and fullness cues. Eat when you're hungry, and stop when you're satisfied, not overly full.

• Avoid Buffets and All-You-Can-Eat Settings: Buffet-style dining can make it challenging to control portion sizes. If dining at a buffet, prioritize nutrient-dense options and use a smaller plate.

• Practice Intuitive Eating: Intuitive eating involves listening to your body and eating based on hunger and fullness cues rather than external rules. This approach can help you maintain a healthy relationship with food.

• Track Your Food Intake: Consider using a food diary or a mobile app to track your meals and portion sizes. This can help you become more aware of your eating habits.

• Be Mindful of Caloric Beverages: Liquid calories from sugary drinks, juices, or high-calorie coffee beverages can add up quickly. Opt for water, herbal tea, or black coffee (without added sugar or cream) during fasting hours.

Remember that portion control is an individualized practice, and what works for one person may not work for another. It may take some time and experimentation to find the portion control strategies that best suit your needs and help you achieve your goals while practicing intermittent fasting.

STRATEGIES FOR STAYING MOTIVATED AND TRACKING PROGRESS WHEN COMBINING INTERMITTENT FASTING WITH THE MIND DIET

Combining intermittent fasting with the MIND diet is a commendable approach to support both your physical and cognitive health. Staying motivated and tracking progress can help you stay committed to this lifestyle change. Here are some strategies to help you stay motivated and monitor your progress effectively:

1. Set Clear Goals:

Define specific, achievable goals related to your health, such as weight loss, improved cognitive function, or better overall well-being. Having clear objectives will give you a sense of purpose and direction.

2. Keep a Journal:

Maintain a journal to track your meals, fasting hours, and how you feel both physically and mentally. Note any improvements in energy levels, cognitive function, or mood.

3. Take Before and After Photos:

Capture images of yourself at the beginning of your journey and periodically thereafter. Seeing visible changes can be a powerful motivator.

4. Monitor Physical Health Indicators:

Keep track of metrics like weight, body measurements, blood pressure, and cholesterol levels. Positive changes in these areas can be a strong indication of progress.

5. Document Non-Scale Victories:

Celebrate small achievements, like having more energy, better concentration, improved sleep, or an increased sense of well-being. These non-scale victories are important markers of progress.

6. Use Technology:

Utilize apps or tools to help track your meals, fasting hours, and physical activity. Many apps can also provide insights into your nutritional intake and progress over time.

7. Establish a Routine:

Creating a consistent routine around your fasting and eating schedule can help reinforce the habit. It becomes part of your daily life rather than an occasional effort.

8. Stay Educated:

Continuously learn about the benefits of both intermittent fasting and the MIND diet. Understanding how these practices positively impact your health can be a strong motivator.

9. Join a Community or Support Group:

Connect with like-minded individuals who are also pursuing similar health goals. Sharing experiences, tips, and successes can be highly motivating.

10. Practice Mindfulness and Gratitude:

Take time each day to reflect on your progress and acknowledge your efforts. Being mindful of the positive changes you're making can boost motivation.

11. Reward Yourself:

Set up a system of rewards for achieving milestones. Rewards can be anything from a new workout outfit to a spa day.

12. Stay Consistent, Not Perfect:

Understand that progress may not always be linear, and that's okay. Aim for consistency in your efforts rather than perfection.

13. Stay Flexible and Adapt:

Be open to adjusting your approach based on how your body responds. What works for one person may not work for another, so listen to your body and make adjustments as needed.

14. Consult Professionals:

Seek guidance from healthcare providers or registered dietitians to ensure that you're on the right track and making progress in a healthy and sustainable way.

Remember that change takes time, and it's important to be patient with yourself. Celebrate your successes, no matter how small, and keep your eyes on the long-term benefits of combining intermittent fasting with the MIND diet for your overall health and well-being.

PART TWO

Spinach and Mushroom Breakfast Quesadilla

Ingredients:

• 1 whole-grain tortilla or flatbread

• 1 cup fresh spinach

• 1/2 cup sliced mushrooms

• 2 tablespoons shredded mozzarella cheese

• 2 tablespoons salsa

Instructions:

1. In a skillet, sauté sliced mushrooms and fresh spinach until wilted.

2. Lay the tortilla flat and sprinkle with shredded mozzarella cheese.

3. Top with the sautéed vegetables and salsa.

4. Fold the tortilla in half and warm in the skillet until the cheese is melted.

Blueberry Walnut Oatmeal

Ingredients:

• 1/2 cup rolled oats

• 1 cup unsweetened almond milk

• 1/2 cup fresh blueberries

• 1 tablespoon chopped walnuts

• 1/2 teaspoon vanilla extract

Instructions:

1. In a saucepan, combine rolled oats and almond milk. Cook until the oatmeal thickens.

2. Stir in fresh blueberries and vanilla extract.

3. Top with chopped walnuts for added crunch and healthy fats.

Avocado and Tomato Breakfast Sandwich

Ingredients:

• 2 slices whole-grain bread, toasted

• 1/2 ripe avocado, mashed

• Sliced tomato and red onion

• 1 poached or fried egg

• Fresh basil leaves for garnish

Instructions:

1. Spread mashed avocado on one slice of toasted bread. Layer with sliced tomato, red onion, and a poached or fried egg.

2. Top with fresh basil leaves and the second slice of toasted bread to make a sandwich.

Coconut and Berry Chia Pudding

Ingredients:

• 2 tablespoons chia seeds

• 1/2 cup coconut milk (canned, unsweetened)

• 1/2 cup mixed berries (strawberries, raspberries, blackberries)

• Unsweetened shredded coconut for topping

• Drizzle of honey (optional)

Instructions:

1. In a bowl or jar, mix chia seeds and coconut milk. Refrigerate for at least 2 hours or overnight.

2. In the morning, layer chia pudding with mixed berries and sprinkle with shredded coconut. Add a drizzle of honey for sweetness if desired.

Peanut Butter and Banana Protein Smoothie

Ingredients:

• 1 ripe banana

• 1 cup unsweetened almond milk

• 1 scoop of your favorite protein powder

• 1 tablespoon natural peanut butter

• Dash of cinnamon

Instructions:

1. Blend banana, almond milk, protein powder, peanut butter, and cinnamon until smooth.

2. Pour into a glass and enjoy your protein-packed smoothie.

Mixed Berry and Almond Overnight Oats

Ingredients:

• 1/2 cup rolled oats

• 1 cup unsweetened almond milk

• 1/2 cup mixed berries (strawberries, blueberries, raspberries)

• 1 tablespoon almond butter

• 1 teaspoon honey (optional)

• Sliced almonds for garnish

Instructions:

1. In a jar or container, combine rolled oats and almond milk. Refrigerate overnight.

2. In the morning, top with mixed berries, almond butter, and a drizzle of honey. Garnish with sliced almonds for added crunch.

Egg and Veggie Breakfast Burrito

Ingredients:

• 2 large eggs, scrambled

• 1 whole-grain tortilla

• Sautéed bell peppers, onions, and spinach

• 2 tablespoons salsa

• Sliced avocado for topping

Instructions:

1. Fill a whole-grain tortilla with scrambled eggs, sautéed veggies, salsa, and sliced avocado.

2. Roll it up to create a breakfast burrito that's both hearty and nutritious.

Greek Yogurt and Berry Parfait

Ingredients:

- 1/2 cup Greek yogurt (low-fat or non-fat)

- 1/2 cup mixed berries (blueberries, strawberries, raspberries)

- 1 tablespoon honey

- Granola for topping (optional)

Instructions:

1. In a glass or bowl, layer Greek yogurt, mixed berries, and honey.

2. If desired, add a sprinkle of granola for added texture and flavor.

Sweet Potato and Black Bean Breakfast Bowl

Ingredients:

- 1/2 cup cooked sweet potato, diced

- 1/2 cup black beans, rinsed and drained

- Sliced avocado

- Salsa or hot sauce for topping

- Poached or fried egg

Instructions:

1. Combine diced sweet potato and black beans in a bowl.

2. Top with sliced avocado, salsa or hot sauce, and a poached or fried egg for extra protein.

Cherry Almond Chia Seed Smoothie

Ingredients:

- 1 cup unsweetened almond milk

- 1/2 cup frozen cherries

- 1/4 cup Greek yogurt

- 1 tablespoon almond butter

- 1 tablespoon chia seeds

• Drizzle of honey (optional)

Instructions:

1. Blend almond milk, frozen cherries, Greek yogurt, almond butter, and chia seeds until smooth.

2. Add a drizzle of honey for sweetness if desired and enjoy your creamy cherry almond smoothie.

Mushroom and Spinach Breakfast Quesadilla

Ingredients:

• 1 whole-grain tortilla

• 1/2 cup sliced mushrooms

• 1 cup fresh spinach

• 2 tablespoons shredded low-fat mozzarella cheese

• 1/4 teaspoon garlic powder

Instructions:

1. In a non-stick skillet, sauté sliced mushrooms until they release their moisture. Add fresh spinach and cook until wilted.

2. Place the tortilla in the skillet and sprinkle with mozzarella cheese. Top with the sautéed mushrooms and spinach. Sprinkle with garlic powder.

3. Fold the tortilla in half and cook until the cheese melts and the tortilla is crispy.

Peach and Almond Breakfast Quinoa Bowl

Ingredients:

• 1/2 cup cooked quinoa

• 1/2 peach, sliced

• 2 tablespoons sliced almonds

• 1/2 teaspoon vanilla extract

• 1 teaspoon honey (optional)

Instructions:

1. In a bowl, combine cooked quinoa, sliced peach, sliced almonds, vanilla extract, and honey (if desired).

2. Stir to combine and enjoy your nutritious quinoa bowl.

Spinach and Tomato Frittata Muffins

Ingredients:

• 4 large eggs

• 1 cup fresh spinach, chopped

• 1/2 cup cherry tomatoes, halved

• 1/4 cup grated Parmesan cheese

• Salt and pepper to taste

Instructions:

1. Preheat the oven to 350°F (175°C).

2. In a bowl, whisk eggs and add chopped spinach, cherry tomatoes, grated Parmesan cheese, salt, and pepper.

3. Pour the mixture into greased muffin cups.

4. Bake for 15-20 minutes or until the frittata muffins are set and lightly browned on top.

Banana and Walnut Breakfast Smoothie

Ingredients:

- 1 ripe banana

- 1 cup unsweetened almond milk

- 2 tablespoons chopped walnuts

- 1 tablespoon honey (optional)

- A pinch of cinnamon

Instructions:

1. Blend banana, almond milk, chopped walnuts, honey (if desired), and a pinch of cinnamon until smooth.

2. Pour into a glass and enjoy your creamy banana walnut smoothie.

Pumpkin and Chia Seed Pudding

Ingredients:

- 2 tablespoons chia seeds

- 1/2 cup unsweetened pumpkin puree

- 1/2 cup unsweetened coconut milk

- 1/2 teaspoon pumpkin spice blend

- 1/2 teaspoon vanilla extract

- A drizzle of maple syrup (optional)

Instructions:

1. In a jar or container, mix chia seeds, pumpkin puree, coconut milk, pumpkin spice blend, and vanilla extract.

2. Refrigerate for at least 2 hours or overnight.

3. Drizzle with maple syrup if you'd like some extra sweetness before serving.

Mediterranean Veggie Omelette

Ingredients:

- 2 large eggs

- 1/4 cup diced tomatoes

- 1/4 cup diced bell peppers

- 1/4 cup chopped spinach

• 2 tablespoons feta cheese

• Fresh basil leaves for garnish

Instructions:

1. Whisk eggs in a bowl and season with a pinch of salt and pepper.

2. Heat a non-stick skillet over medium heat and add a bit of cooking spray.

3. Pour the whisked eggs into the skillet and cook until set. Add diced tomatoes, bell peppers, spinach, and feta cheese on one half of the omelette.

4. Fold the other half over the veggies, cook for another minute, and garnish with fresh basil.

Cherry Almond Breakfast Quinoa

Ingredients:

• 1/2 cup cooked quinoa

• 1/4 cup unsweetened almond milk

- 1/4 cup dried cherries

- 1 tablespoon chopped almonds

- 1 teaspoon honey (optional)

Instructions:

1. In a bowl, combine cooked quinoa, almond milk, dried cherries, chopped almonds, and honey (if desired).

2. Stir well and enjoy your hearty quinoa bowl.

Smoked Salmon and Dill Cream Cheese Bagel

Ingredients:

- 1 whole-grain or whole-wheat bagel

- 2 tablespoons light cream cheese

- 2 oz smoked salmon

- Fresh dill and lemon zest for garnish

Instructions:

1. Toast the bagel until lightly browned. Spread cream cheese on each bagel half.

2. Layer with smoked salmon, fresh dill, and a sprinkle of lemon zest.

Banana and Spinach Green Smoothie

Ingredients:

• 1 ripe banana

• 1 cup unsweetened almond milk

• 1 cup fresh spinach leaves

• 1 tablespoon almond butter

• 1/2 teaspoon honey (optional)

Instructions:

1. Blend banana, almond milk, fresh spinach, almond butter, and honey (if desired) until smooth.

2. Pour into a glass and enjoy your nutrient-packed green smoothie.

Greek Yogurt and Berry Stuffed Crepes

Ingredients:

- 2 whole-grain or whole-wheat crepes

- 1/2 cup Greek yogurt (low-fat or non-fat)

- 1/2 cup mixed berries (blueberries, raspberries, strawberries)

- 1 tablespoon honey

Instructions:

1. Lay the crepes flat and spread Greek yogurt on each.

2. Top with mixed berries and drizzle with honey.

3. Roll up the crepes and enjoy your delightful breakfast.

Salmon and Avocado Salad

Ingredients:

• 4 oz grilled or baked salmon

• 1/2 avocado, sliced

• Mixed greens (arugula, spinach, romaine)

• Cherry tomatoes, halved

• Lemon-Dill Vinaigrette (mix olive oil, lemon juice, fresh dill, salt, and pepper)

Instructions:

1. Arrange mixed greens on a plate and top with grilled salmon, avocado slices, and cherry tomatoes.

2. Drizzle with Lemon-Dill Vinaigrette for a refreshing salad.

Mushroom and Lentil Soup

Ingredients:

• 1 cup cooked green or brown lentils

- 8 oz mushrooms, sliced

- 1/2 cup diced onions

- 2 cloves garlic, minced

- 4 cups vegetable broth

- 1 teaspoon thyme

- Salt and pepper to taste

Instructions:

1. In a large pot, sauté diced onions and minced garlic until translucent.

2. Add sliced mushrooms and cook until they release their moisture.

3. Stir in cooked lentils, vegetable broth, thyme, salt, and pepper.

4. Simmer for 15-20 minutes, allowing the flavors to meld together.

Greek-Style Quinoa Bowl

Ingredients:

• 1 cup cooked quinoa

• Sliced cucumber and red onion

• Kalamata olives

• Feta cheese

• Hummus for dipping

• Tzatziki sauce (optional)

Instructions:

1. In a bowl, combine cooked quinoa, sliced cucumber, red onion, Kalamata olives, and crumbled feta cheese.

2. Serve with a side of hummus for dipping and tzatziki sauce, if desired.

Tofu and Vegetable Stir-Fry

Ingredients:

• 4 oz tofu, cubed

• 2 cups mixed stir-fry vegetables (broccoli, bell peppers, snap peas)

• 2 tablespoons low-sodium soy sauce or teriyaki sauce

• 1/2 teaspoon ginger, minced

• 1/2 teaspoon garlic, minced

Instructions:

1. In a skillet, stir-fry tofu and mixed vegetables until tender.

2. Add low-sodium soy sauce or teriyaki sauce, minced ginger, and minced garlic.

3. Stir to combine and cook for an additional 2-3 minutes.

Caprese Quinoa Salad

Ingredients:

• 1 cup cooked quinoa

• Cherry tomatoes, halved

• Fresh mozzarella balls

• Fresh basil leaves

• Balsamic glaze and olive oil for drizzling

• Salt and pepper to taste

Instructions:

1. In a bowl, combine cooked quinoa, cherry tomato halves, fresh mozzarella balls, and fresh basil leaves.

2. Drizzle with balsamic glaze and olive oil. Season with salt and pepper.

Mediterranean Quinoa Salad with Chickpeas

Ingredients:

• 1 cup cooked quinoa

• 1 can (15 oz) chickpeas, drained and rinsed

• 1/2 cucumber, diced

• 1/2 cup cherry tomatoes, halved

• 1/4 cup red onion, finely chopped

- Kalamata olives, pitted and sliced

- Feta cheese crumbles

- Lemon-oregano dressing (olive oil, lemon juice, dried oregano, salt, and pepper)

Instructions:

1. In a large bowl, combine cooked quinoa, chickpeas, cucumber, cherry tomatoes, red onion, Kalamata olives, and feta cheese.

2. Drizzle with the lemon-oregano dressing and toss to combine. Serve chilled.

Lentil and Spinach Stuffed Sweet Potatoes

Ingredients:

- 2 medium sweet potatoes

- 1 cup cooked green or brown lentils

- 1 cup fresh spinach leaves

- 1/4 cup diced red bell pepper

- 1/4 cup crumbled goat cheese

- Balsamic glaze (optional)

Instructions:

1. Pierce sweet potatoes with a fork and microwave until tender.

2. Slice the sweet potatoes open and fluff the insides.

3. Stuff each sweet potato with cooked lentils, fresh spinach, diced red bell pepper, and crumbled goat cheese.

4. Optionally, drizzle with balsamic glaze before serving.

Thai-Inspired Tofu Salad

Ingredients:

- 4 oz extra-firm tofu, cubed and pan-fried

- Mixed greens (romaine lettuce, spinach, cilantro)

- Shredded carrots

- Sliced bell peppers

- Edamame beans (steamed)

- Thai peanut dressing (peanut butter, soy sauce, lime juice, honey, and sriracha)

Instructions:

1. Arrange mixed greens on a plate and top with pan-fried tofu, shredded carrots, sliced bell peppers, and edamame beans.

2. Drizzle with the Thai peanut dressing for a flavorful salad.

Cauliflower Rice and Shrimp Stir-Fry

Ingredients:

- 4 oz shrimp, peeled and deveined

- 2 cups cauliflower rice

- 1 cup mixed stir-fry vegetables (broccoli, snap peas, bell peppers)

- Low-sodium soy sauce or teriyaki sauce

- 1/2 teaspoon ginger, minced

- 1/2 teaspoon garlic, minced

Instructions:

1. In a skillet, stir-fry shrimp and mixed vegetables until the shrimp turn pink.

2. Add cauliflower rice, low-sodium soy sauce or teriyaki sauce, minced ginger, and minced garlic.

3. Stir to combine and cook for an additional 2-3 minutes.

Greek Chickpea Wraps

Ingredients:

• Whole-grain or whole-wheat wraps

• 1 can (15 oz) chickpeas, drained and mashed

• Chopped cucumber, tomato, and red onion

• Fresh parsley

• Tzatziki sauce

Instructions:

1. Lay the wraps flat and spread a layer of mashed chickpeas.

2. Top with chopped cucumber, tomato, red onion, fresh parsley, and a drizzle of tzatziki sauce.

3. Roll up the wraps and enjoy your Greek-inspired meal.

Spinach and Berry Salad with Grilled Chicken

Ingredients:

• 4 oz grilled chicken breast, sliced

• Baby spinach leaves

• Mixed berries (strawberries, blueberries, raspberries)

• Sliced almonds

• Balsamic vinaigrette dressing (olive oil, balsamic vinegar, Dijon mustard, honey)

Instructions:

1. Arrange baby spinach leaves on a plate and top with grilled chicken slices, mixed berries, and sliced almonds.

2. Drizzle with balsamic vinaigrette dressing for a vibrant and nutritious salad.

Vegetable and Lentil Curry

Ingredients:

• 1 cup cooked green or brown lentils

• Mixed vegetables (bell peppers, zucchini, carrots)

• 1 can (14 oz) diced tomatoes

• 1 can (14 oz) light coconut milk

• Curry powder, turmeric, and cumin to taste

• Fresh cilantro for garnish

Instructions:

• In a pot, sauté mixed vegetables until tender.

• Stir in cooked lentils, diced tomatoes, light coconut milk, and spices.

• Simmer for 15-20 minutes until the flavors meld together.

• Garnish with fresh cilantro and serve with brown rice.

Greek Quinoa and Chickpea Bowl

Ingredients:

• 1 cup cooked quinoa

• 1 can (15 oz) chickpeas, drained and rinsed

• Diced cucumber, red onion, and tomato

• Kalamata olives

• Crumbled feta cheese

• Greek dressing (olive oil, red wine vinegar, oregano, garlic, salt, and pepper)

Instructions:

1. In a bowl, combine cooked quinoa, chickpeas, diced cucumber, red onion, tomato, Kalamata olives, and crumbled feta cheese.

2. Drizzle with Greek dressing and toss to combine.

Broccoli and Cheddar Stuffed Baked Potatoes

Ingredients:

• 2 medium russet potatoes, baked

• 1 cup steamed broccoli florets

• 1/2 cup shredded sharp cheddar cheese

• Greek yogurt or sour cream (optional)

• Chopped chives for garnish

Instructions:

1. Cut baked potatoes open and fluff the insides.

2. Stuff each potato with steamed broccoli and shredded cheddar cheese.

3. Optionally, add a dollop of Greek yogurt or sour cream and garnish with chopped chives.

Asian-Inspired Tofu and Vegetable Salad

Ingredients:

• 4 oz extra-firm tofu, cubed and pan-fried

• Mixed greens (romaine lettuce, spinach, arugula)

- Sliced bell peppers

- Sliced cucumber

- Sliced scallions

- Sesame ginger dressing (sesame oil, rice vinegar, soy sauce, honey, ginger)

Instructions:

1. Arrange mixed greens on a plate and top with pan-fried tofu, sliced bell peppers, cucumber, and scallions.

2. Drizzle with sesame ginger dressing for an Asian-inspired salad.

Miso-Glazed Salmon with Quinoa and Steamed Broccoli

Ingredients:

- 4 oz salmon fillet

- 1 cup cooked quinoa

- Steamed broccoli florets

• Miso glaze (miso paste, soy sauce, mirin, brown sugar, grated ginger)

Instructions:

1. Preheat the oven to 400°F (200°C).

2. Brush salmon with miso glaze and bake for 12-15 minutes until cooked.

3. Serve with cooked quinoa and steamed broccoli.

Chickpea and Kale Sauté with Lemon and Garlic

Ingredients:

• 1 can (15 oz) chickpeas, drained and rinsed

• Fresh kale leaves, chopped

• 2 cloves garlic, minced

• Zest and juice of 1 lemon

• Red pepper flakes (optional)

• Olive oil for sautéing

Instructions:

1. In a skillet, sauté minced garlic in olive oil until fragrant.

2. Add chickpeas and kale, and sauté until kale is wilted.

3. Drizzle with lemon zest, lemon juice, and red pepper flakes (if desired).

Tomato and Basil Quinoa Risotto

Ingredients:

• 1 cup cooked quinoa

• Cherry tomatoes, halved

• Fresh basil leaves, chopped

• 1/4 cup grated Parmesan cheese

• Olive oil

• Balsamic glaze for drizzling

Instructions:

1. In a pan, sauté cherry tomatoes in olive oil until they soften.

2. Stir in cooked quinoa and fresh basil leaves.

3. Serve with grated Parmesan cheese and a drizzle of balsamic glaze.

Spicy Black Bean and Veggie Wrap

Ingredients:

• Whole-grain or whole-wheat wrap

• 1 cup black beans (canned, drained, and rinsed)

• Sliced bell peppers, onions, and zucchini

• Sliced jalapeños (optional)

• Greek yogurt or sour cream (optional)

Instructions:

1. Lay the wrap flat and spread a layer of black beans.

2. Top with sautéed sliced bell peppers, onions, and zucchini.

3. Add sliced jalapeños for extra spice and a dollop of Greek yogurt or sour cream (optional). Roll up the wrap and enjoy.

Ingredients:

• 1 can (5 oz) tuna, drained and flaked

• Cherry tomatoes, halved

• Cucumber slices

• Kalamata olives

• Red onion, thinly sliced

• Feta cheese crumbles

• Lemon vinaigrette (olive oil, lemon juice, Dijon mustard, oregano)

Instructions:

1. In a bowl, combine flaked tuna, cherry tomatoes, cucumber slices, Kalamata olives, red onion, and feta cheese.

2. Drizzle with lemon vinaigrette for a Mediterranean-inspired salad.

Vegetarian Sheet Pan Fajitas with Mushrooms and Peppers

Ingredients:

Fajita Seasoning

- 2 tsp chili powder

- 2 tsp ground cumin

- 2 tsp Mexican oregano

- 1 tsp smoked paprika

- 1 tsp Kosher salt, more to taste

- Fresh ground black pepper, to taste

Fajitas

- 4 Portabello mushrooms caps, sliced

- 2 bell peppers (red and orange) cut into strips

- 1 red onion, slices into wedges

- 3 cloves garlic, sliced

• 3 Tbs olive oil

• ¼ cup chopped fresh cilantro leaves

• 2 limes (1 for juicing, 1 to serve as wedges)

• 8 small corn or flour tortillas, warmed or toasted over open flame

• 2 avocados

Instructions:

1. Preheat oven to 400° F. Lightly coat a large sheet pan with non-stick spray.

2. In a small bowl, combine chili powder, cumin, Mexican oregano, paprika, 1 tsp salt and a few grinds of pepper.

3. Spread sliced mushrooms, bell peppers, onion and garlic onto the prepared baking sheet. Sprinkle chili powder mixture over the veggies. Drizzle olive oil over the top and gently toss to coat the veggies.

4. Place into oven and bake for 20 minutes.

5. Before serving, squeeze the juice of 1 lime over entire sheet pan and toss.

6. Serve immediately with tortillas. Top with cilantro, guacamole and extra diced red onion and lime wedges.

Tahini Noodle Bowl with Edamame

Ingredients:

• 1 red pepper, diced

• 1 cup frozen edamame, steamed (you can steam them in their pods or already shelled – whatever you find in your grocery store)

• 6 green onions, chopped

• Sesame seeds, to garnish

• 5 oz brown rice + millet Ramen noodles, cooked (2 noodles cakes)

Tahini – Peanut Butter Dressing

• 1 Tbs tahini

- 1 Tbs peanut butter

- 1 Tbs extra-virgin olive oil

- 1 garlic clove, minced

- 1 Tbs fresh lime juice

- 1 Tbs rice vinegar

- 2 tsp Sriracha

- 2 Tbs warm water, more as needed

- ½ tsp Kosher salt

- ¼ tsp honey

Instructions:

1. Steam edamame in a large stock pot with steamer basket. (I use frozen edamame in pods and remove the pod after steaming, approx. 10 minutes until tender).

2. Season with a couple pinches of salt after cooking.

3. In a small Cuisinart or blender, mix all tahini dressing ingredients until emulsified.

4. Cook noodles according to package instructions. Drain and rinse.

5. Chop the red pepper and scallions. Place in a large bowl.

6. Add steamed edamame, noodles and tahini sauce. Taste and adjust for salt.

7. Add sesame seeds to top + serve with extra Sriracha and a lime wedge.

Maple Pecan Granola with Olive Oil

Ingredients:

• 3.5 old-fashioned rolled oats

• 1 cup hulled raw pumpkin seeds

• 1 cup hulled raw sunflower seeds

• 1 cup unsweetened coconut chips

• 1 ¼ cups raw pecans left whole or coarsely chopped

• ¼ cup ground flax seed

• ¼ cup wheat germ (optional)

- ½ cup pure maple syrup

- ½ cup extra-virgin olive oil

- 1/3 cup coconut sugar or packed light brown sugar

- 1 tsp coarse salt

- Serve over Greek yogurt and top with fresh berries

Instructions:

1. Heat oven to 300°F.

2. Place oats, pumpkin seeds, sunflower seeds, coconut, pecans, flax, wheat germ, maple syrup, olive oil, sugar, and 1 teaspoon salt in a large bowl and mix until well combined. You'll need to mix it well to evenly coat everything with the wet ingredients.

3. Spread granola mixture onto a rimmed baking sheet lined with parchment paper. Transfer to oven and bake, stirring every 10 to 15 minutes, until granola is toasted, about 45 minutes.

4. Remove granola from oven and let cool. Stores up to one month in an airtight container.

5. Serve over Greek yogurt and fresh berries.

Berry Spinach Salad with Maple-Balsamic Vinaigrette

Ingredients:

- 6 cups baby spinach (or any super green combo)

- 1 cup any combo of blueberries and/or blackberries

- 1/3 cup sliced almonds, toasted

- Feta cheese, crumbled to top (optional)

- A sprinkle of hemp seeds, to top (optional)

Maple-Balsamic Vinaigrette

- ¼ cup extra virgin olive oil

- 2 tsp balsamic vinegar

- 1 tsp Dijon mustard

- 1 Tbs maple syrup

- Salt and fresh ground pepper, to taste

Instructions:

Maple-Balsamic Vinaigrette

1. Combine all ingredients in a mixing bowl; whisk until well combined and thoroughly incorporated.

Berry Spinach Salad

1. Toast almonds in a dry pan over medium-low heat. Careful to watch them so they don't burn! Set aside.

2. In a large bowl, lightly toss spinach with a couple tablespoons of dressing. You want a super light coating on the greens. You'll most likely have some dressing left over.

3. Add in berries and gently toss again. Top with toasted almonds and a light drizzle of additional dressing.

Mulligatawny Soup

Ingredients:

- 4 Tbs olive oil

- 1 large Spanish onion, chopped

- 6 cloves garlic, finely chopped

- 3 Tbs fresh ginger, finely chopped peeled

- ½ jalapeño, stemmed, seeded, and chopped

- 1 Tbs ground coriander

- 2 tsp ground cumin

- 1 ½ tsp ground turmeric

- 1 ½ cups red lentils

- 8 cups vegetable or chicken broth

- 3 Tbs minced cilantro leaves

- 1 cup unsweetened canned coconut milk

- ¼ cup freshly squeezed lemon juice

- 2 tsp kosher salt

- Freshly ground black pepper

- Dukkah, to top

Instructions:

1. Heat the olive oil in a large pot over medium-high heat. Add the onion, garlic, ginger, and jalapeño and cook, stirring, until browned, about 12 minutes.

2. Lower the heat to medium, stir in the coriander, cumin, and turmeric, cook until fragrant, stirring, for 45 seconds.

3. Pour in the broth and bring to a boil. Add the lentils, lower the heat and simmer, covered, until very tender, about 30 minutes.

4. Remove from heat. Stir in the cilantro and salt.

5. Working in batches, transfer the mixture to a blender and puree until smooth, or puree with an immersion blender. Return the puree to the pot and reheat over medium heat.

6. Whisk in the coconut milk (keep some aside to make a pretty swirl on top), lemon juice, and season with salt and pepper to taste.

7. Serve immediately with cilantro and nutty dukkah topping, if desired.

Vegan Broccoli Salad with Couscous, Raisins + Almonds

Ingredients:

• 2 tablespoons olive oil

• ½ yellow onion, diced

• 1 tsp curry powder

• 2.5 cups chopped broccoli (bite-sized pieces)

• 3 cloves garlic, chopped

• 15 oz canned chickpeas, rinsed + drained

• 1/3 cup golden raisins

• 1.25 cup water (divided)

• ¾ cup dry couscous

• Kosher salt

• ½ lemon, juice only

• 1/3 cup sliced almond, toasted

• Harissa paste, to taste

Instructions:

1. In a large saucepan, heat the oil over medium-high heat.

2. Add chopped onion. Season with a few pinches of salt and pepper. Sauté 3-4 minutes until starting to soften.

3. Add curry powder. Stir to incorporate.

4. Add chopped broccoli, another couple pinches of salt and ¼ cup water. Cook over medium-high heat, tossing occasionally, until tender, 2 to 3 minutes.

5. Stir in garlic, chickpeas, raisins, 1 cup water, and ½ teaspoon salt. Bring to a boil.

6. Stir in the couscous, cover, and remove from heat. Let steam 5 minutes, then fluff with a fork.

7. Mix in fresh lemon juice.

8. Top with toasted almonds. (Dry toast them over medium heat on the stove top for 3-4 minutes until starting to brown.)

9. Serve with harissa paste + additional lemon wedge. Add more salt and pepper to taste.

Vegan Buddha Bowls with Roasted Cauliflower

Ingredients:

• 1 head cauliflower (about 4 – 5 cups chopped)

• 12 baby potatoes, sliced in half length-wise

• 6 cups chopped curly kale

• 1 recipe chipotle mayo sauce (you'll use about half)

• 2 Tbs avocado or olive oil

• Salt + pepper

• Creamy Chipotle Dressing

Pesto Sauce (optional)

• 2 cups fresh spinach (or any greens)

• 3 Tbs pine nuts (or walnuts)

• 1 large garlic clove, crushed

• Salt + pepper

• 3 Tbs olive oil

Instructions:

1. Preheat oven to 400F.

2. Cut cauliflower into small florets. Place in small bowl. Toss with avocado oil, salt and pepper.

3. Slice potatoes in half lengthwise. Place in small bowl. Toss with avocado oil, salt and pepper.

4. Place cauliflower and potatoes on separate rimmed baking sheets lined with parchment. This parchment paper is reusable!

5. Add ¼ cup of water to each rimmed baking sheet.

6. Cover each baking sheet tightly with foil. The extra water steam the veggie first – making them soft and tender.

7. Bake for 15 minutes. Remove foil.

8. Bake for another 30 minutes until tender and starting to brown.

9. About 5 minutes before the potatoes and cauliflower are done roasting, sauté the kale in a little olive oil, just until starting to wilt.

10. Toss roasted potatoes with pesto, if using.

11. Divide all veggies between bowls. Top with chipotle dressing.

Pesto Sauce

1. In a small Cuisinart, blend nuts, garlic, salt and pepper.

2. Once a grainy paste forms, add spinach. Pulse until all spinach is chopped into tiny bits.

3. Add olive oil, 1 Tbs at a time, until pesto is emulsified. Taste + add additional salt + pepper if needed.

Shaved Brussels Sprout Salad with Pistachios + Honey Vinaigrette

Ingredients:

For the Honey Vinaigrette:

• 3 Tbs honey

• ¼ cup apple cider vinegar or white wine vinegar

• 6 Tbs extra virgin olive oil

- ¾ tsp Kosher salt

- ¼ tsp black pepper

For the Salad:

- 1.5 lbs raw brussels sprouts

- 1 cup toasted pistachios, lightly salted (I like a mix of whole pistachios + crushed in this salad)

- 1 cup shaved parmesan or pecorino romano

- Salt and pepper to taste

- Optional: ½ cup shaved red onion

Instructions:

For the Honey Vinaigrette:

1. Place all ingredients together in a mason jar and shake until emulsified. Or use a small Cuisinart and blend.

For the Salad:

1. Shave brussels sprouts

2. Toss with honey vinaigrette.

3. Add pistachios and parmesan. Optional red onion. Toss again.

4. Add salt and pepper to taste.

Creamy Wild Rice and Mushroom Soup

Ingredients:

• 1 cup uncooked wild rice blend

• 4-5 cups fresh cauliflower florets (usually 2 small organic cauliflower heads)

• 2/3 cup raw cashews

• 1 ½ cups water

• 2 tablespoons fresh lemon juice

• 2.5 tablespoons olive oil

• 3 stalks celery, diced (about 1 cup)

• 1 cup shallots, finely diced (about 2 large)

- 4 large cloves garlic, minced

- 4 cups vegetable broth

- 16 oz sliced mushrooms, white or baby portabella

- 2 Tbs fresh thyme, chopped (divided)

- 2 teaspoons Kosher salt (divided)

- Freshly ground black pepper to taste

Instructions:

1. Cook wild rice (I use Lundberg Wild Rice blend) according to package instructions. Drain and set aside. Approx. 45 min to cook.

2. While cooking the rice, start on the cauliflower, mushrooms and shallots/celery mixture.

CAULIFLOWER CASHEW CREAM

1. Place a steam basket in a large pot, add an inch or 2 of water to the bottom, steam cauliflower florets with the lid on, medium to medium-high, until extremely fork tender. Approx. 10 min. Drain and transfer to blender.

2. In a high-speed blender, add water, cashews, lemon juice, and 1.5 tsp Kosher salt. Add steamed cauliflower. Blend on high (liquid setting on a Vitamix) until completely smooth and creamy. Approx. 2-3 min. Set aside until ready to mix cashew cauliflower cream into soup.

MUSHROOMS

1. In another sauté pan, add 2 tsp olive oil over medium-high heat. Add mushrooms and 1 Tbs chopped thyme. Cook until mushrooms have taken on color, 5- 10 minutes, stirring occasionally. Once cooked, season with ½ tsp kosher salt. Set aside until ready to add to soup.

SHALLOTS/CELERY/GARLIC

1. In a large stockpot, add 2 Tbs olive oil.

2. Over medium heat, sauté shallots, celery, and 1 Tbs. thyme. Sprinkle with a few pinches of salt and a few grinds of the pepper mill. Sauté for about 5 minutes, or until the vegetables just begin to soften, stirring occasionally.

3. Add the garlic and cook for an additional minute.

4. Stir in the vegetable broth. Keep this stockpot warm (low heat) and covered until your rice is done cooking in the other pot.

5. Once rice is ready, add rice, sautéd mushrooms and cauliflower cashew cream to the stockpot. Stir gently to combine.

6. Increase the heat to medium-low and continue to simmer covered for just 5 minutes or until soup is hot and ready to enjoy!

7. Season with Kosher salt and black pepper to taste. Sprinkle each bowl with extra thyme. Enjoy!

Pear Salad with Arugula, Manchego + Roasted Pepitas

Ingredients:

- 1 5 oz mixed baby spinach and arugula

- 1/3 cup pepitas, lightly toasted

- 5 oz Manchego cheese, sliced paper thin

- 2 large Bartlett pears, sliced into thin strips

Salad Dressing

- 1/3 cup olive oil

- 3 Tbsp sherry vinegar or apple cider vinegar

- 1 tsp honey

- 1 tsp grainy mustard

- ¼ tsp Kosher salt

Instructions:

Salad Dressing

1. Add all ingredient to a small Cuisinart and blend until emulsified. Or add to a glass jar with lid and shake vigorously until emulsified. Set aside.

Salad

1. In a small skillet, add 2 tsp olive oil over medium-low heat. Add pepitas and toss until coated with olive oil. Sprinkle with salt and continue stirring, roasting until just starting to brown. Be careful – sometimes pop they! Approx. 3 minutes.

2. Toss greens with a light coating of salad dressing. If not serving right away, wait to dress the greens. *NOTE: There will be extra salad dressing.

3. Layer with slices of pears, Manchego and top with toasted pepitas.

Sweet Potato Hash Bowl with Cilantro Pesto

Ingredients:

• 4 cups sweet potato, peeled and diced

• 4 cup red beets, peeled and diced

• 1 tsp Kosher salt

• 2 Tbsp olive oil

• 4 eggs, cooked to your preference

• 1 15 oz can garbanzo beans, drained and rinsed (optional instead of eggs)

• 2 large avocados

Cilantro Pistachio Pesto

- ¼ cup pistachios (other nuts, such as cashews, can be used)

- 1.5 cups cilantro, packed (leaves and stems)

- 1/3 cup olive oil

- Juice of ½ of a lime

- 1-3 Tbsp water

- ¼ tsp Kosher salt

Instructions:

1. Heat oven to 400F.

2. Each in separate bowls, toss diced beets, sweet potatoes and chickpeas (if using) with 1 Tbsp olive oil and a couple generous pinches of kosher salt.

3. Roast beets and sweet potatoes separately on rimmed baking sheets until edges are browning. Veggies should take 25 – 30 minutes. If using chickpeas, do the same process except they'll take about 15 minutes.

4. Toss each halfway through.

5. While the vegetables are roasting, cook eggs to your preference to top the hash bowls.

6. After the veggies are roasted, distribute them between four bowls. Top with an egg, sliced avocado and drizzled with Cilantro Pesto sauce.

Cilantro Pistachio Pesto

1. Pulse cilantro and pistachios in a high speed blender or Cuisinart until chopped into small bits.

2. Add in remaining ingredients EXCEPT water and blend until a smooth sauce is formed. Add 1 Tbs of water at a time if the sauce is too thick.

Mushroom Tacos with Spicy Kale and Feta

Ingredients:

Portabello Mushrooms

• 4-5 large portabello mushroom caps, sliced thick

• 1 tsp red wine vinegar

• 1 clove garlic, crushed

• 1 Tbs parsley, chopped

Kale

• 4 cups curly kale, stems removed and chopped into bite sized pieces

• 1 Tbs olive oil

• 3 tsp adobo sauce

• ¼ tsp chili powder

• 1 tsp Kosher salt, divided

Toppings, Etc.

• 1 pint cherry tomatoes, sliced in half

• Feta, crumbled (to top)

• Flour tortillas, browned on each side (I use whole wheat tortillas)

Instructions:

Kale:

1. Trim the kale and place in a large mixing bowl.

2. Add 1 tablespoon of olive oil, 3 tsp adobo sauce, ¼ tsp chili powder and ¼ tsp salt. Toss it all together and use your hands to massage the ingredients into the kale. Set aside.

Portabello Mushrooms:

1. Slice mushrooms and place in over medium heat in a sauté pan. I don't usually add any olive oil as the mushrooms will release liquid as they cook.

2. Once they are tender (5-6 minutes), turn off the flame and toss with red wine vinegar and crushed garlic. Then toss with chopped parsley and season with salt and pepper to taste.

Taco Assembly:

1. Brown each tortilla over an open flame. Too much and they will be crispy, so just enough to get a little char in places. This can be started while the mushrooms are cooking.

2. Load tortilla with a scoop of kale and a couple slices of mushrooms.

3. Top with cherry tomatoes and feta.

Beet & Chickpea Salad with Coconut Lime Dressing

Ingredients:

Coconut Lime Dressing

• ½ cup fresh cilantro leaves rinsed and packed (plus more to top salad)

• 1.5 tbsp fresh lime juice; zest the lime first and set aside

• 4 tsp white balsamic vinegar apple cider vinegar or rice wine vinegar

• ½ cup light coconut milk

• 1 Tbsp coconut oil melted

• 1 Tbsp maple syrup

• ¼ tsp kosher salt plus more to taste

Salad

• 4-5 medium red beets roasted, peeled and chopped (about 4-5 cups)

• 1 cup cooked chickpeas rinsed and drained (use more if desired)

• 1 lime grated zest

Instructions:

Dressing

1. Add all dressing ingredients to a Cuisinart and blend until emulsified.

Salad

1. In a large bowl, mix the chopped beets with the dressing.

2. Add chickpeas and extra cilantro, toss gently.

3. Top with reserved grated lime zest and extra lime wedges

Baked Salmon with Garlic-Butter Asparagus

Ingredients:

• 4 oz salmon fillet

• Asparagus spears

- 1 clove garlic, minced

- 1 tablespoon butter

- Lemon wedges

- Fresh dill for garnish

Instructions:

1. Preheat the oven to 400°F (200°C).

2. Place salmon on a baking sheet and season with salt, pepper, and minced garlic.

3. Bake for 12-15 minutes until salmon flakes easily.

4. In a separate oven-safe dish, roast asparagus with a drizzle of olive oil, salt, and pepper until tender.

5. Serve salmon and asparagus with a pat of butter, lemon wedges, and fresh dill.

Mushroom and Spinach Stuffed Chicken Breast

Ingredients:

- 2 boneless, skinless chicken breasts

- Fresh spinach leaves

- Sliced mushrooms

- 1 clove garlic, minced

- 1/4 cup grated Parmesan cheese

- Olive oil for sautéing

Instructions:

1. Preheat the oven to 375°F (190°C).

2. Butterfly each chicken breast and stuff with fresh spinach, sliced mushrooms, minced garlic, and grated Parmesan cheese.

3. Sear the stuffed chicken breasts in a hot skillet with olive oil until golden.

4. Transfer to the oven and bake for 20-25 minutes until the chicken is cooked through.

Quinoa and Roasted Vegetable Bowl

Ingredients:

- 1 cup cooked quinoa

• Roasted vegetables (bell peppers, zucchini, cherry tomatoes)

• Chickpeas, roasted or canned

• Tahini dressing (tahini, lemon juice, garlic, water)

Instructions:

1. In a bowl, combine cooked quinoa, roasted vegetables, and chickpeas.

2. Drizzle with tahini dressing for a hearty and flavorful bowl.

Shrimp and Broccoli Stir-Fry

Ingredients:

• 4 oz shrimp, peeled and deveined

• Broccoli florets

• Sliced bell peppers

• 1/2 cup snap peas

• Stir-fry sauce (soy sauce, honey, ginger, garlic)

Instructions:

1. In a skillet, stir-fry shrimp, broccoli, sliced bell peppers, and snap peas until shrimp turn pink and vegetables are tender.

2. Drizzle with stir-fry sauce and serve over brown rice.

Eggplant and Chickpea Curry

Ingredients:

• 1 medium eggplant, diced

• 1 can (15 oz) chickpeas, drained and rinsed

• Diced tomatoes (canned or fresh)

• Curry powder, cumin, and turmeric to taste

• Coconut milk

• Fresh cilantro for garnish

Instructions:

1. In a pot, sauté diced eggplant until slightly browned.

2. Add chickpeas, diced tomatoes, and spices. Simmer until the eggplant is tender.

3. Stir in coconut milk and simmer for an additional 5 minutes.

4. Garnish with fresh cilantro and serve with rice or quinoa.

Lemon Herb Grilled Chicken with Quinoa and Roasted Vegetables

Ingredients:

• 4 oz grilled chicken breast, marinated with lemon juice and fresh herbs

• 1 cup cooked quinoa

• Roasted mixed vegetables (carrots, bell peppers, red onion)

• Fresh parsley for garnish

Instructions:

1. Grill chicken until cooked through and infused with lemon and herbs.

2. Serve alongside cooked quinoa and a side of roasted vegetables.

3. Garnish with fresh parsley.

Mediterranean Stuffed Bell Peppers

Ingredients:

• 4 bell peppers, halved and seeds removed

• Ground turkey or lean ground beef

• Cooked quinoa

• Chopped tomatoes, cucumber, and red onion

• Feta cheese crumbles

Instructions:

1. In a skillet, brown ground turkey or beef and mix with cooked quinoa, chopped tomatoes, cucumber, red onion, and feta cheese.

2. Stuff each bell pepper half with the mixture and bake at 375°F (190°C) for 25-30 minutes until peppers are tender.

Teriyaki Tofu and Broccoli Stir-Fry

Ingredients:

• 4 oz extra-firm tofu, cubed and pan-fried

- Broccoli florets

- Sliced bell peppers

- Teriyaki sauce (low-sodium)

- Steamed brown rice

Instructions:

1. In a skillet, stir-fry pan-fried tofu, broccoli florets, and sliced bell peppers with low-sodium teriyaki sauce.

2. Serve over steamed brown rice.

Cauliflower and Chickpea Curry

Ingredients:

- 1 small cauliflower, cut into florets

- 1 can (15 oz) chickpeas, drained and rinsed

- Diced tomatoes (canned or fresh)

- Curry spices (turmeric, cumin, coriander)

- Coconut milk

- Fresh cilantro for garnish

Instructions:

1. In a pot, sauté cauliflower florets until lightly browned.

2. Add chickpeas, diced tomatoes, and curry spices. Simmer until cauliflower is tender.

3. Stir in coconut milk and simmer for an additional 5 minutes.

4. Garnish with fresh cilantro and serve with brown rice or whole-grain naan.

Lentil and Spinach Stuffed Bell Peppers

Ingredients:

- 4 bell peppers, halved and seeds removed

- 1 cup cooked green or brown lentils

- Fresh spinach leaves

- Diced tomatoes

- Italian seasoning

• Mozzarella cheese (optional)

Instructions:

1. Preheat the oven to 375°F (190°C). Steam fresh spinach until wilted.

2. Mix cooked lentils with diced tomatoes and Italian seasoning. Stuff each bell pepper half with lentil mixture and a layer of spinach.

3. Optionally, top with mozzarella cheese. Bake for 25-30 minutes until peppers are tender and cheese is melted.

CONCLUSION

In combining intermittent fasting with the MIND diet, you embark on a journey towards optimizing both your physical and cognitive well-being. This dual approach holds immense promise, as it leverages the benefits of time-restricted eating alongside a diet rich in brain-boosting nutrients. By strategically timing your meals and embracing the principles of the MIND diet, you not only enhance your metabolic health but also nurture your cognitive function and potentially reduce the risk of neurodegenerative diseases.

Portion control and mindful eating become the cornerstones of this endeavor, allowing you to savor nutrient-dense foods while maintaining balance. By being attuned to your body's cues and making deliberate choices, you foster a sustainable lifestyle that supports your health goals. Furthermore, tracking your progress through journals, measurements, and technological aids not only provides tangible evidence of your journey but also serves as a source of motivation and reinforcement.

The synergy between intermittent fasting and the MIND diet is underscored by their shared emphasis on whole, unprocessed foods. This partnership culminates in a lifestyle that not only promotes physical vitality but also nurtures cognitive resilience. The scientific foundations underpinning these approaches lend credibility to their potential benefits, offering a solid rationale for their adoption.

However, it's crucial to approach this combined approach with mindfulness and flexibility. Bodies and lifestyles vary, and what works for one individual may require adaptation for another. Consulting with healthcare professionals or registered dietitians can provide personalized guidance, ensuring that your chosen path aligns harmoniously with your unique health needs.

Ultimately, as you navigate the realms of intermittent fasting and the MIND diet, remember that progress is a journey, not a destination. Embrace each milestone, both big and small, and cultivate a spirit of self-compassion. By embracing this comprehensive approach to health, you embark on a transformative voyage towards a more vibrant and resilient version of yourself.